Hot & Sexy

Hormone Solution

By George F. Moricz, M.D.

© 2017 George F. Moricz, M.D.

TABLE OF CONTENTS

Acknowledgments

It is with great appreciation that I thank all of the doctors and patients who made me rethink everything I ever learned and taught me the importance of becoming a student again.

INTRODUCTION

For the first time, interviewers can steal a "sneak peek" into the stunning breakthrough known as the ***Hot & Sexy Hormone Solution based on Dr. Moricz' revolutionary Youthful Blueprint System™***.

This sought-after system is no surprise to his many clients who have been endlessly raving about their life-changing transformations. No longer are they agonized by memory lapses, fatigue, aging before their time, sleep issues or weight gain because there is now a simple certainty of tapping into the benefits of *youthfulness* quicker than they ever dreamed possible with this proven solution.

Before you commit to another product, pill or supplement, or purchase another gym membership, or book another doctor's visit, STOP and devour every page of this must-read book to avoid the humiliation and misery of not knowing your ***hormonal blueprint.*** Join the smart and select few who already have the bragging rights of knowing their hormonal blueprint, today!

FREE GIFTS TO HELP YOU!

- **Take Dr. Moricz' Beauty Quiz and receive your custom skin blueprint results! www.skinblueprint.com**

- **Take Dr. Moricz' Sleep Quiz and Discover *How to go from Sleep Deprived to* Sleeping Beauty: www.mybodyhormone.com**

- **Discover New Secrets to Weight Loss: www.loseweightnow.solutions**

THE REASON FOR THIS BOOK

In medicine, we are often told that our patients are our greatest teachers. I couldn't agree more. That is one of the reasons why I have undertaken the task of writing this book—to share with you the valuable lessons I have learned from my own patients. In fact, one patient in particular is largely responsible for the book you hold in your hands today. Without him showing up in my practice with a series of puzzling medical issues, none of this probably would have happened.

My aim in writing the *Hot & Sexy Hormone Solution* is to describe to you a medical program that has taken me more than ten years to develop, fine tune, apply, test, and share comfortably with proven results with people from all walks of life.

First, let me begin with a description of the individual who forced me to rethink everything I had ever learned in medical school and specialty training in order to address a critical problem. People may or may not realize that as a medical student, one is often forced to explain to professors the real reason for doing something. Later, as a fully trained doctor, I had to research the real reason that the following person's problem was not being improved with everything available in a first-world culture of medicine in the United States. After sorting through mounds and mounds of information over thousands of hours, I came to a very real conclusion that most of what I had been taught, and seen in literature really didn't work for this individual. I will also share that for a very special reason, I will not disclose the identity of the person until later in this book.

Let's first start with a description of the individual…

A man in his early thirties came to me with a history of not sleeping well for six years. Despite changes in work schedule, eating and lifestyle habits, which had also included specific sleep habits, there was unfortunately no improvement. In summary, he reported poor, interrupted sleep that left him drawn and unrefreshed in the morning. By afternoon, he experienced the most exhausting fatigue. His immune function had been compromised, and he was getting ill more often. He also had difficulty absorbing food, and experienced multiple food intolerances and weight loss. All in all, he lost much of the enjoyment of life due to all of these problems.

After implementing, over the course of a year, what is now known as the *Hot & Sexy Hormone Solution using the Youthful Blueprint System™,* this individual regained not only restful sleep, but renewed daytime energy and improvements in body composition, including muscle and loss of fat, and began to rebuild his immune system. Basically, you might say that he started enjoying life again with a "refreshed outlook."

This is why I'm writing this book—not to describe what one person overcame, but to describe what one person made me *rethink about everything that I'd been taught and had been convinced incorrectly was the proper approach to helping people with problems just like his.*

Now you may still be asking, what is the real purpose in undertaking this type of book for the benefit of other people?

My aim is to divulge a lifetime's treasure trove of secrets based not only on critical observations supported by science, but *"real results"* and transformations for scores of people. That's the real reason.

As an aside, in a world with heavy advertising and promotions, an important message can be lost in the mix of before-and-after photos, unreproducible testimonials and the latest fads. Internet and continuous TV advertising, and trial/error approaches can be made to look like "the real deal." But let me just say that the pages you are about to read are meant to rid you of a life of trial and error.

Because what is the reality of life? It's really about time. But for many people, it is time without results. As a word of advice, investing in your time correctly by making it count is probably the biggest take-home message this book offers. But where do you turn to get the most out of time? We're in a world where everything costs you—when what you thought you would receive in return for value has not yielded the net. And that really is a cost. So, wouldn't it make sense to have a system that rids you of trial and error, and finally allows you to make better use of your time?

Now, as a warning, some of the things that you will read in this book will shock you, contradict what you've been told, make you feel foolish, and maybe even make you feel as though you have been duped. Once you overcome this, however, then and only then will you be able to tap into the very secrets contained within each chapter. I will also make you this promise—the true identity of the individual previously described will be disclosed. Not for the purposes for making this book more important, but to show you how sometimes human effort can be swayed by necessity. In other words, many people have benefitted from this system, but it's only because someone had suffered from the lack of such a system that it could be made possible.

Since you are still reading at this point, it is evident that your openness to hearing what is about to be said will allow you to benefit greatly. Once again, there are many who would never even take this step, and therefore will remain in a trial-and-error mode for the rest of their lives.

So congratulations for your perseverance in finding the solution to your hormone challenges and difficulties. Let's get started…

WHAT CLIENTS ARE SAYING

This is what Dr. Moricz' Clients are saying…

"Dr. Moricz is an angel in a doctor's suit. I am certain of this! I thank God every day for Dr. Moricz and his staff. The way that I feel now is totally opposite of how I felt walking into his office the first time:

- I have lost twenty-eight pounds in two months.
- I have no more hot flashes.
- My energy level is great!
- I sleep through the night.
- I don't sleep until 3 p.m. every day
- My depression has gone away.
- I am happy again.
- Sex with my husband is better than it has ever been in my life! Imagine that!

"I am loving life! This whole process has been a miracle in my life. I am fifty-six years old and feeling the way I did when I was twenty!" —E.B., female, age fifty-six

"I am a stage IV cancer survivor, who was suffering from severe fatigue due to chemo, radiation, and multiple surgeries. I feel so blessed to have found Dr. Moricz and his staff. His treatments have definitely helped me regain strength when nothing else worked. You're an answer to my prayers, Dr. Moricz. Keep on helping people. Your work is deeply appreciated and thoroughly worthwhile." —P.P., female, age fifty-four

"I visited my dermatologist yesterday. They asked me for an update on meds I was taking. Ha! There were about ten on the list. I smiled as I drew a line through all except a couple of supplements. It felt great. This program is very comprehensive. Dr. Moricz has shown me how to rebuild the energy and vitality that I lost when I hit my fifties. So many old aches and pains have either diminished or disappeared completely. For years, I went to bed tired and woke up tired. Over the past few weeks, I've noticed that after six or so hours of rest, I'm ready to go.

In addition, I had a procedure three years ago that nearly took my life. It left me with intense pain in my feet, legs, and forehead. Now I go days at a time without noticing discomfort.

Thank-you doctor for your research and dedication to finding a more natural pathway to health and healing."
—B.E.

"Over thirty years ago, I was a Middle-Eastern belly dancer. Thank God for Dr. Moricz' wonderful BODY HORMONE BALANCE PROGRAM. I am dancing again with the grace and beauty of this art form at age sixty-seven. My limbs are flexible; once again I can go down to the floor and come back up gracefully. I feel great and youthful again. LIFE IS GOOD." —W.D.

"I lost thirty pounds of fat and gained ten pounds of muscle, when no other diet or weight loss program produced lasting results. I have the energy and stamina to work out consistently and have improved mental focus. Please pray for my wife because my libido is off the chart!" —J.H.D.

"I began with Dr. Moricz in February 2010. My health had bottomed out, and I desperately needed help that conventional doctors had not given me. Most of my issues are weight-related. I lost forty pounds in four months, and even after getting off the program after eight months, I still manage to keep most of it off." — K.S.

"This program was a lifesaver for me. When I started the program, I had no energy and weighed almost 400 pounds. Now, I walk four miles a day, and can easily walk across the room without getting out of breath. If you need to lose weight, please give this program and Dr. Moricz a chance to make you healthy." —T.W.

"I didn't realize how bad I actually felt until I felt this good! My sleep has improved, my energy levels have improved, and my ability to focus has improved. I'm not HOT all the time! This is BY FAR, the best thing I have ever done for myself. My husband also told me to let the staff know that if they needed a testimonial from him on how this has drastically improved his life, he would be happy to give you one also! Love it! Love it! Love it!" —K.J.

"The Body Hormone Balance Program has restored my sex drive. I even look at my husband differently. My youth is back, and so is my sense of well-being, happiness, enthusiasm and energy. I'm also ready to take on new challenges. I could go on and on. Thank you for restoring all in my life." —R.J.

"Dr. Moricz and his staff have given me a new start on life, and have basically retrained me in my eating habits. The program has made all the difference in the world. I feel better and have more energy than I have had in years." —D.B.D

LIVES. CHANGED.

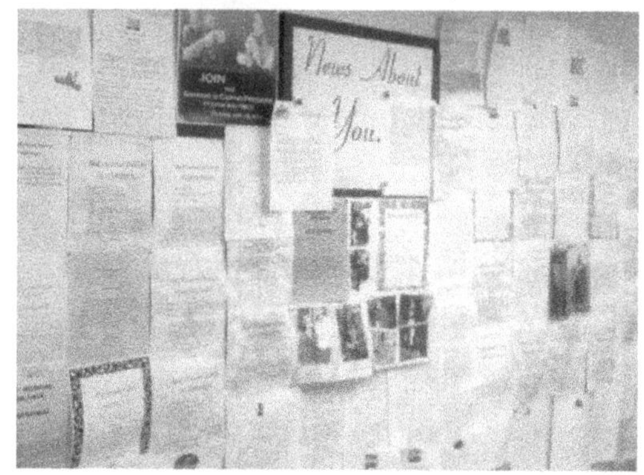

George F. Moricz, MD
Founder of Your Youthful Blueprint

Click below to preview some of the amazing success stories shared by Dr. Moricz's clients who rave about his Youthful Blueprint System –

www.beautychannelmd.com

FUN FACTS ABOUT DR. MORICZ:

- His father was an engineer who designed super highways. Dr. Moricz worked for his father doing blueprints to make money during school; his mother is from Central Europe and introduced him to high living standards of beauty and lifestyle.

- Two thirds of Dr. Moricz' new clients are family and friends of existing clients.

- Dr. Moricz has what he calls the "30-day rule". 'Your partner will come to see me because they will not be able to keep up with you.' (*Clients being treated in program).

- Dr. Moricz' staff is worried for his safety and what the public will think because Dr. Moricz relentlessly takes on the medical establishment (doctor clinics, pharmaceutical industry, and insurance companies) to protect the health of his clients.

- Dr. Moricz is straight shooter and does not sugarcoat the truth.

- V.I.P. clients are happiest even though Dr. Moricz is very expensive, and they don't mind because of the incredible results they receive.

- A number of Dr. Moricz' clients pre-order products before Dr. Moricz even carries them in his office.
- Clients who have been coming to Dr. Moricz on a continual basis never miss his live events.
- Dr. Moricz hates waiting in lines; Dr. Moricz hates government and insurance companies; Dr. Moricz loves exotic cars.
- Dr. Moricz does not sugarcoat the truth; he is strict but fair.

PERSONAL HISTORY:

- Dr. Moricz lived in small town where a Midwest doctor named Doctor Jenkinson was his family doctor who subconsciously influenced Dr. Moricz to take care of people one on one.
- Dr. Moricz was almost disabled by exhaustion. Dr. Moricz had to rethink everything he ever learned in medical school.
- Dr. Moricz discovered a breakthrough to save himself from exhaustion (known as the Youthful Blueprint System™). Dr. Moricz "cracked the code" with this blueprint system

because his dad was an engineer and always told him to go back to the blueprint when things were wrong.

- Dr. Moricz invented a breakthrough sleep system known as Dr. Moricz' Ultimate Sleep Solution™ for which he is now the manufacturer. This system saved him from sleep deprivation which he suffered for over six years.

- This sleep system gets most of his patients the sleep they need because it is an all-natural system and supplement that is customized to their sleep brain chemistry. This has never been done this way before.

- Dr. Moricz developed a breakthrough beauty solution called the "Exclusive European Rejuvenator System" which has a guarantee to take ten years off your face in less than 10 days and comes with a money back guarantee. He developed this system because women in his family twisted his arm and said "Come on, you can do this…you have custom-designed many things."

CHAPTER 1: DESIGNING SUCCESS

I feel compelled to share a story that caught me 'off guard' and gave me a perspective that helped me understand something more valuable than what I thought I was really doing.

A pretty sharp lady made a confession to me—so here it goes....

Before she made the decision to come to me on the quest to get back her life, she felt like she was going to amateurs   -- she had every imaginable health care advisor, expert and doctor OFFER her BIG short term promises that would fix everything ... what she painfully realized (after losing lots of time, money and quality years) is that she was in the little leagues by going to technicians and mechanics WHEN instead she should have started with me "because <u>you are reengineering my body</u> <u>and mind</u> NOT just changing or throwing parts at me *like a car.* Because of this approach, I witnessed my productivity and relationships transform themselves literally overnight <u>which is what I was really looking for in the first place</u>..."

Shared by one of my VIP clients, she nailed down a principle that has become more strikingly clear to other clients as well…

YOUR BODY AND MIND WERE ENGINEERED FOR YOUTH

Why am I sharing this and why now?

In a moment, I will share a story of what made me do what I do today. For many years, I had many people come to me looking for their youthful blueprint. Twenty years as a doctor I *finally* 'cracked the code' on youth with three seldom shared but very potent secrets:

ACCEPTED FACT #1: Youth is perfect health. In other words, when you had youth it didn't matter if you slept right, ate right, you woke up the next day, you had lots of energy and you certainly didn't have sexual trouble.

ACCEPTED FACT #2: When you had youth, you had the perfect combination of natural chemicals and hormones running through your brain and body.

ACCEPTED FACT #3: When I rewind you back to your youthful blueprint, you start enjoying all the things you ONCE enjoyed about being young again.

When you had youth, you not only *had* the perfect combination of natural chemicals and hormones but it is this very perfect combination of these natural hormones and chemicals that *gave you youth --* which is your youthful blueprint – the SECRET basis of every transformation enjoyed by my clients.

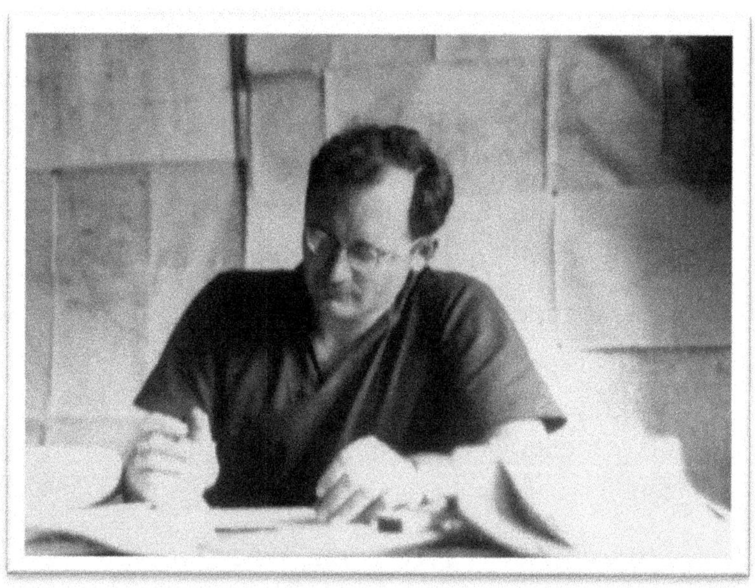

A PHOTO OF MY FATHER DESIGNING SUPERHIGHWAYS

SO what was the <u>real influence</u> as to why a doctor surgeon who was trained in traditional principles *risk everything and would* exit the comfort and convenience of a well-established medical practice, to design a superior approach for re-engineering (designing YOU back) what was perhaps the most perfect thing about you – your youthful blueprint?

It was my father.

My father was a structural engineer who dedicated himself to designing superhighways for much of his career. I grew up influenced by engineering principles which ONLY many years later critically became a 'game changing breakthrough' for my work in helping people as a doctor. But most critical of all, what I discovered was that there was a huge advantage to having grown up as the son of an engineer with exposure to the design of highways, bridges and very impressive structures.

More specifically, the concept of designing *blueprints* would later be the very breakthrough and perhaps the greatest medical breakthrough that I had witnessed as a doctor. See, if my father had been a medical doctor, I would probably have stayed within the box of usual conventional approaches. But the very day that I asked myself *"Why is it that doctors are constantly treating people with the assumption that they should be sick and come to the doctor sick and will ultimately stay sick and BELIEVE that they were never really youthfully healthy in the first place ...?"*

In fact, they did have a time in their life when they had perfect health and that's what we call youth. Then I started to wonder, "What if I could take people back to this perfect combination of youthful chemicals and hormones and give them back all the things they enjoyed about being young again ...?"

Well, over time all these questions volcanically collided together and created a lot of controversy with what doctors and everyday people are taught. The one thing that was hard to argue with were RESULTS of enjoying your youthful blueprint -- the life changing results that people enjoyed in their relationships, energy and ability to enjoy life the way they did years ago but now at a point in their life with acquired experience that time has given them as well.

So, it was my father's influence that made me think of **designing blueprints**. In my teenage years, I worked doing engineering drafting and *blueprints* for my father and *only many years later* did I fully appreciate how there was an *undiscovered blueprint* that everybody was walking around with but very few people were enjoying (until now of course). That's why I believe discovering your unique custom blueprint is perhaps one of the greatest discoveries of medical science, and I am glad to have created this system to share for 'smart and savvy people' who come to me from all over the country.

In a recently released book *Applied Minds: How Engineers Think* by Guru Madhaven, the author says that engineers have been recognized as heroes in designing everything like our: iPhone, microprocessors, computer codes, pharmaceuticals, rockets, electrical systems and air traffic control. More specifically, the "golden basis" to all these engineering marvels is three separate but equally unifying principles:

> **First**: Good engineers create *structures* so they can understand - pre-emptively - the context and value of any given problem and solution.

> **Second**: After that, they acknowledge *constraints* whether of money or politics or available materials, that they must work within or somehow supersede.

> **Third**: They deftly evaluate *trade-offs* so that they can formulate the most effective application for a given situation.

So, you may already be wondering WHY is it that so many people who are *fortunate to discover their very own youthful blueprint* 10, 20, 30 years since they were actually youthful YET "still stay stuck" UNNECESSARILY even though they do not have to?

The ANSWER for this is the very reason that they could not transform their productivity, relationships and lead a very BIG LIFE in the first place:

THEY ARE STUCK IN NON-ENGINEERING PRINCIPLES

In the left-handed box **(figure 1)** below they have been told so many times over and over again and have erroneously convinced themselves that they should start searching for a solution of constraints evaluating trade-offs, limitations and self-doubt to seal and almost guarantee failure.

The success of using sound engineering principles can be summarized in a 3-step model as noted in **figure 2**. The first principle of designing an engineering structure comprehensively matches the underlying problem with a solution. It is the first and only step taken first. It is only after this first step is developed that the second principle of constraints, be it money, preference or truly defined limitations are applied to the first principle of a structured problem-solution. Then, the third engineering principle of evaluating trade-offs so that the most effective application can be formulated for a given situation.

Most people arrive to me "STUCK" in the left-handed column approach:

Figure 1 – One Step model.

In most cases, they have never been shown the successful 3-step engineering model of designing a success blueprint. So, they are continuously and religiously "STUCK" in a One-Step non-engineered approach that has already compromised their chances of success for a very BIG LIFE.

(Figure 1)
Aging before your time

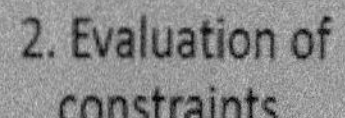

(Figure 2)
Look, feel, and perform li
you did in your twenties

So, how can you "IMMEDIATELY benefit from the secret" that took me twenty years to discover as a Doctor and a lifetime of learning from my father so that you, too, can now lead a very BIG LIFE with supercharged relationships and productivity RIGHT NOW ...

Discovering the above 3-step principles for designing success is perhaps your key to unlocking everything that I have helped you discover with your youthful blueprint. In other words, the most fortunate of people even when given their youthful blueprint (who are "stuck" in a non-engineered one step principle) shown in **figure** 1 will never fully enjoy the benefits of their youthful blueprint.

On the other hand, with a healthy sense of skepticism by opening your mind to a 3-step engineering design for success **(figure 2)** applied to your individualized youthful blueprint practically guarantees your odds for success.

Let me warn you - time and time again there are those who are given their blueprint, who stare at their blueprint, who acknowledge that it exists, who wish to think differently about their blueprint, and delay the inevitable only to eventually realize that *"facts are stubborn things"* – the quicker, the sooner that you take action on rediscovering your youthful blueprint saves years of frustration and puts you light years ahead for taking years off your age even when nothing else has never worked. Now, you have the golden key for how I can re-engineer success with your youthful blueprint so you can now enjoy all the things that you once enjoyed about being young again. There is only power in action so stop delaying any further.

Look, feel, and perform like you did in your 20's in record time even when nothing has ever worked.

Be a "spy on the wall" and discover why Dr. Moricz' VIP Clients never miss any of his "LIVE" events:

www.beautychanneldoc.com

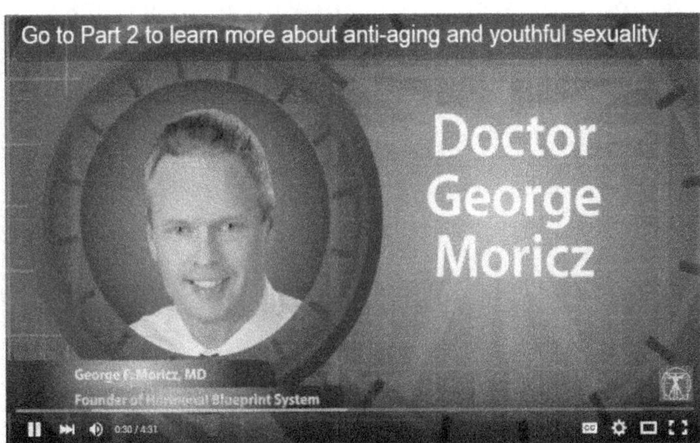

Chapter 2: Youth is Perfect Health

Let's take a moment to look back at when you were twenty years of age. That's right. Rewind back to your 20-year-old image of yourself. Remember how you felt? Remember how you looked? Remember the energy you had, and how you looked forward to every day? When you were 20 years old, you didn't have to eat right, and you didn't have to sleep right. You woke up feeling great nearly every day, and you certainly didn't have any sexual trouble.

This is the basis for the *Hot & Sexy Hormone Solution* and my custom designed *Youthful Blueprint System™*. In other words, you have a 20-year-old blueprint. And with this blueprint that you had at 20, you had possibly the best profile of hormonal balance and nutrition than you would ever have in your life. Had I met you when you were 20, I would have analyzed your weight and body composition; I would have analyzed your hormonal levels; I would have analyzed your intracellular nutrition and performed a functional assessment of your health. Then, later in life, when you decided that things weren't going so well, another assessment would be performed, measuring, once again, weight and body composition and hormonal and nutritional profiles, along with a functional assessment of your health.

Then, comparisons would be made and re-adjustments would be recommended.

Imagine if you will that an architect has the blueprints for a building. Then over time, with shifts in land, as well as settling of the house and the wear and tear on the structure of the building, a reassessment would have to be made to return things to the original blueprint. Well, this is no different than returning you to your 20-year-old blueprint.

When clients come to me in their late 20's and early 30's, they may be experiencing a nosedive in their hormones. Half the people I see with no symptoms at all actually demonstrate changes at the level of the ***cell and blood hormones***, which are already starting the eventual nosedive of perfect hormonal balance and nutritional protection they once enjoyed.

However, what is more common in conventional medicine is to wait until men and women are well into their 40's and 50's and beyond before intervening.

People are all too familiar with the terms **MENOPAUSE** and **ANDROPAUSE**. This chapter will not spend time arguing the exact definitions and whether there is complete hormonal cessation in men and women. But what is important is the timing of the intervention. In other words, what is the benefit of waiting until there is a complete nosedive in hormones and nutrition when someone has chronologically aged, rather than attacking the issue well before health problems arrive?

What is all this talk about *hormones*, what are we really trying to measure? When speaking about hormones, important categories include:

- Reproductive hormones

- Stress gland hormones

- Thyroid hormones

- Pancreatic hormones.

Other non-hormonal measurements, which are interrelated, include **body composition**, which specifically looks at the amount of muscle and fat in the body.

It is well known that when people are aging before their years, they not only have changes in cognitive function, a decrease in energy, an increase in fatigue, but also an increase in weight, and, in particular, a decrease in muscle and an increase in fat.

In twenty years, the standard of care is likely to involve an analysis of body composition, where the fifth vital sign will include measurement of body fat percentage. In other words, people will not only know their blood pressure, pulse, temperature and weight, but they will also know their body fat percentage. **A lot could be said about this, but for practical purposes, knowing body fat percentage is already signifying the early signs of inflammation in the body and hormonal imbalance**.

So, what are people doing to address this, and what is the medical profession recommending?

Well, we all know that people will use caffeine, stimulants and any over-the-counter fix, including the use of sugar, to help them fix issues with energy, focus and metabolism. When the individual actually seeks medical help, it is not uncommon to be placed on stimulants for focus and weight control. It is not uncommon to be prescribed antidepressants and sedatives to help mood and coping issues with daily life, and it is not uncommon to be prescribed sleep aids to help with disruptive sleep.

By the time somebody reaches age 50, the medical establishment is well-versed in the use of synthetic hormones for diagnoses such as **MENOPAUSE** and **ANDROPAUSE**. It is beyond the scope of this book to cover the pros and cons of these approaches, but mentioning them brings attention to the fact that "this" is the usual chronology.

I would suggest that, whether it is over-the-counter or prescribed, that intervention should start between the ages of 30 and 50 when strides can be made, and not in the 50+ age category after a lot of ground has already been lost.

Let's talk about some of the mechanisms of aging.

Everywhere you turn, you hear about "healthy aging," or "anti-aging." Just for a point of reference, there are a number of different mechanisms that have been proposed to stop the aging process, including reversing damage from free radicals, inflammation, insulin resistance and mitochondrial dysfunction. Put simply, there are molecules called free radicals that require neutralization so they don't cause damage. There are chemicals related to inflammation that are spewed from everything from fat cells all the way to the breakdown of certain ingested foods. Still further, there is the issue of pre-diabetes, which eventually can manifest itself as full diabetes. And finally, there are energy powerhouses within the cells called mitochondria, which, as they become less efficient, are associated with loss of energy.

What we are discussing here could be summed up as the diagnosis for aging.

In addition, many times, people are told that, because they are aging, there is a corresponding drop in their hormones. It is not to suggest that the nosedive in hormones described earlier is responsible for every seen and unseen hidden ill of aging. But what if the hormonal nosedive were responsible at some level for the aging process, as well?

Let me suggest it another way: Consider, if you would, that many medical problems that people are experiencing may not really be true medical problems at all! They may be a function of hormonal imbalance.

The number and different types of hormones may not be particularly important to list, identify, and write about in this short book. However, consider that, whenever hormones are not in the perfect blueprint ratio that was present in your 20's, your body may be in hormonal imbalance. Once again, as you age, there is an association with decreased hormones. So, what if the decrease in hormones is the cause of aging and all its unpleasant side effects inside and outside of your body?

A WORD OR TWO ABOUT HORMONES. Hormones as chemical messengers serve many critical functions. The body is often considered a balance of the breakdown and buildup of tissues for proper functioning. Words such as *"anabolic"* versus *"catabolic"* are often used. Think of anabolic as rebuilding and protecting your body and catabolic as breaking down tissues, especially during signs of inflammation. So in essence, what if hormones could regulate inflammation? There is a field called immunomodulation which essentially focuses on hormones, particularly the male-derived ones that are involved with regulation of inflammation. This actually makes a lot of sense, because you notice that as you get older you are often plagued with immune and inflammatory problems, which you were able to handle much easier earlier in life.

A WORD OR TWO ABOUT NUTRITION

Earlier, these chemicals, called free radicals, were mentioned. They are responsible for cell damage and are probably heightened during exercise and while eating. Nutritional supplementation and properly balanced antioxidants with foods are thought to be protective. Nutrition is also important when looking at energy. Earlier, I mentioned *mitochondria*, which are the powerhouses within cells. It is now thought that in muscles, and to a degree in the brain, that these powerhouses may be the connection not only for energy, but the protection of the cell's longevity. So, it makes sense to see nutrition from a cell protective perspective, as well as an energy perspective, as well.

No discussion would be complete without a brief word on environmental exposures…

Everywhere you turn, you will see information on everything from toxic metals, and chemicals in the environment. It is thought that, both at the level of damaging cells, as well as disrupting hormonal balance in the body, that environmental exposure is responsible for everything from infertility, some cancers and shortened lifespan.

A holistic approach would argue that many people do not recover from traditional medical approaches because removal of these toxic exposures has not been complete. While I cannot exclude the possibility of this, it arguably makes sense to optimize hormonal balance to assist the body in helping it repair itself and improve its immune function. Certainly, as the body ages, it has to deal further with cell damage and repair.

Another perspective on aging is that it is the breaking down of most processes into inflammation and energy issues. Think about inflammation as removing offending agents in the body so that rebuilding of the tissues can occur. This can explain in simple terms everything from allergies to autoimmune diseases (i.e., rheumatoid and lupus).

With respect to energy, the brain and the body depend on proper powerhouse function so that there can be an efficient processing of nutrition to make a currency we now know as ATP. Based on breakdown of the particular processes that are involved in the transfer of nutrients and co-factors, it is evident that nutrition is critical for energy production within the cell.

***So what does anti-aging have to do with all this*? Nutrition and hormonal balance are the most effective ways to attack inflammation and energy issues.**

On the surface, one could evaluate body composition, skin and hair quality, and sexual function. On a deeper level, hormones and nutrition affect the immune system. An entire field of *immunomodulation* has been built on the role of hormones regulating the immune system.

Nutrition is equally important, especially when it comes to looking at foods and seeing how they affect anti-inflammatory pathways in the body. In summary, the ***Hot & Sexy Hormone Solution using the Youthful Blueprint System™*** is based on complete balance of all of your hormones.

Hormones can work with or against each other, which is why hormonal expertise in balancing these hormones as correlated with symptoms is performed on an individual basis. Put another way, you have a 20-year-old blueprint for both nutrition and hormones.

When it comes to handling illnesses involving issues with energy and inflammation, it is critical in the experience of this system to return an individual to the 20-year-old blueprint so that the body can best handle the processes that are causing the problem.

As an example, in conventional medicine, when people come in with issues of energy, a common culprit is the use of statin medications, which are used to attack cholesterol abnormalities. As another example, the medications used for chemotherapy and rheumatoid arthritis are often so toxic to regular cells, that they can over-suppress the immune system and make one susceptible to basic infections. Still others receive medications including corticosteroids (commonly known as the prednisone-type medications) which can also suppress the immune system, strip the body of bone and muscle, and cause elevations in blood sugar and blood pressure, if left unchecked.

One has to wonder—once most people return to their 20-year-old blueprint, how much less dependence on prescription medication and how much less disability they would have to deal with if they received this approach, rather than the conventional one?

In the next several chapters, I'd like to take some time to educate you about the *Hot & Sexy Hormone Solution using the Youthful Blueprint System™*. First off, it's based on the balancing of hormones. This approach is used to attack weight issues, fatigue issues, and many other basic problems, including depression, anxiety, sleep disruptions and poor coping, through a more structured approach.

Once again, think back to how you felt when you were twenty. Remember how you dealt with weight issues, coping issues and day-to-day stresses when you were in complete hormonal balance? You probably dealt with these issues a lot differently than you do today. In the coming chapters, I look forward to sharing more insight into the Hormone Blueprint System with you, since *youth is perfect health*.

Chapter 3: Weight Issues

The following are a *collection of interview questions* asked during expert consultations with Dr. Moricz. They have been arranged for ease of reading.

Interviewer: Dr. Moricz, just to remind our audience that two thirds of the adults in the United States are either overweight or obese and, furthermore, there is an unprecedented rise in childhood obesity. Is this really the fault of the American public?

Dr. Moricz: There certainly are cultural and attitude issues toward eating, exercise and weight control. However, from the 1970s and 1980s, the American Diabetes Association took a position on carbohydrates [sugars] that probably contributed more to the rise of diabetes and obesity. More specifically, it was decided prematurely that low-fat diets would be superior to the current dietary recommendations of the time. What this meant was that more than 50 percent of calories would be derived from carbohydrates, or sugar, to create a low-fat diet. It has been shown through weight management studies that low-fat diets have higher failure rates than almost any other type of diet. And for the purposes of our discussion, by encouraging increased carbohydrate consumption, the American Diabetes Association provided the seeds for the rise in overweight and obese adults.

Interviewer: So, are you in favor of restricting carbohydrate sugars?

Dr. Moricz: Well, first it's important to define that there are different types of sugars [carbohydrates] that have different assigned glycemic load and glycemic index values.

Glycemic index and glycemic load reflect how the body's blood sugar will react when different types of these sugars are eaten. So basically, these numbers will give information to people concerned about causing unnecessary sugar elevations in their blood by helping them choose carbohydrates that are less likely to do that. Just as important is looking at other factors that may affect blood sugar levels as well.

First, fiber is extremely important since this might reduce the spike of the sugar after the carbohydrate is ingested. Next, the relative ratio of protein to carbohydrates will often determine how much of an insulin response is necessary to handle the sugar while still achieving appetite suppression. Still, the beneficial use of fats in a diet may actually help reduce the spike in sugar that would be much higher if a person were not to use any fat at all. So, essentially, what is being asked is, ***"What is a 'hormonal' approach to weight management?"*** This is based not on calorie counting, but on what certain foods do to hormones, such as insulin. There are different ways of thinking about this, but consider this—there is a way to eat daytime meals that only minimally elevates necessary insulin levels three times a day—if at all. Put differently, there is a way of structuring an eating plan that may not require the body to elevate insulin markedly through the day and, therefore, avoid the regular effects of insulin on fat storage, while allowing stored sugar molecules to be used for energy burning.

Interviewer: So, are you focusing on hormones like insulin?

Dr. Moricz: That's right. I realized that whatever system was developed for weight control was really being designed to prevent pre-diabetes and stop worsening of existing diabetes, depending on the person. See, burnout of the pancreas—an organ producing several hormones including insulin—occurs with the consistent carbohydrate challenge, i.e., the typical Standard American Diet (S.A.D.). So when the American Diabetes Association, medical societies and government agencies encouraged increasing carbohydrates in the 1970s and the 1980s, they were, in fact, promoting what we call *insulin resistance.*

Interviewer: We hear a lot about the connection between diabetes and early aging. Would you comment on this?

Dr. Moricz: There are different ways to explain this, but think of the body's poor handling of sugar that results in damage to many cells within the body through a process called *glycation.* Therefore, when a person has syrupy blood, or "too much sugar," sugar is deposited into many cells including nerves and blood vessels, causing damage. One of the ways that the body prematurely ages is by challenging it with too much sugar carbohydrates.

Let's look at it another way. First, too much sugar challenge will overwork the insulin production of the pancreas, which eventually causes burnout of the pancreas.

Secondly, without adequate insulin at the right time [when eating carbohydrates], then sugar levels rollercoaster which forces a person to increase carbohydrate intake because sugar cannot reliably be driven into the body's cells at the right time. So, all of this excessive sugar converts into fat. Insulin has some beneficial role in delivering sugar and amino acids, which are the building blocks of protein, into cells, however, it also promotes fat formation, which is stored as body fat, or as a fatty liver. Ultimately, the continued deposits of sugar into the nerves and blood vessels causes damage which clinically is seen as an increased rate of heart attacks and damage to the kidneys and eyes, among other well-known complications of diabetes. In other words, diabetes accelerates the aging process.

Interviewer: What is the advantage of catching diabetes early?

Dr. Moricz: Look at how many people who are already suffering with diabetes may also have issues with weight control as well. Increased body fat weight is really a symptom of early insulin resistance, or pre-diabetes. That's why attacking weight management from a hormonal approach is the ONLY logical approach to me that is based on solving the original problem.

Interviewer: That's interesting. Dr. Moricz, then do you suspect that is the reason that so many undiagnosed pre-diabetics are showing up at your office with weight control issues?

Dr. Moricz: You nailed it on the head. Aging can be a combination of several processes going wrong. For example, the hormonal changes that a body will undergo as early as the 20's and 30's reflects aging unless it is attacked at the onset.

Interviewer: So, maybe when people say, "You are getting older and your hormones are changing," really what they mean is, "Because your hormones are changing, you are starting to get older"?

Dr. Moricz: Indeed. And I think medicine has really missed the boat on helping people lose weight. And by that, I mean body fat weight.

Interviewer: How so?

Dr. Moricz: For starters, look around at how many commercial programs there are like the ones advertised on TV, print media and the Internet and ask yourself, "Are they really founded on sound principles?"

Interviewer: Tell me more. Does calorie counting really work?

Dr. Moricz: That's an excellent question, and I'm glad that you brought that up. There are really two important definitions that must be covered to understand anything else I am going to say. And these are the two critical definitions: LCD (low-calorie diet) and VLCD (very-low calorie diet). LCD is an 800-1,200 calorie diet. VLCD is a 400-800 calorie diet. So a low-calorie diet is often what you see advertised in the media. A very-low calorie diet is a restrictive diet recommended by doctors who practice bariatrics.

These are doctors dedicated to the study of weight management and involved in close supervision of people on these diets. Commercial programs are designed to be low-calorie diets. For purposes of our discussion, restricting calories alone will never increase metabolism and may actually slow metabolism in the long run. A second flaw about counting calories is using weight as the only outcome. All weight tells you is that you are on the Earth and not on the moon. If I wanted to decrease your weight, I would send you to the moon and weigh you. The most important concept that invariably keeps people in the dark is "focusing on weight alone and not body composition."

Interviewer: Interesting, Dr. Moricz. Then how do you account for your success with the *Hot & Sexy*

Hormone Solution using your Youthful Blueprint System™? How do you teach your clients and get the success that your system is well known for?

Dr. Moricz: You brought up a valid point and I will share the secret that has enabled people to go from measuring a number that is not essentially as important as the next concept that I'm going to discuss, which is body composition. In other words, how do you show people the value of switching from measuring weight to actual body composition so that their success is better monitored and long-term success can even be achieved?

Well, let me start with a very simple example. Take Arnold Schwarzenegger, whom most people know from either the movies or politics, or just from living in the United States. Take someone of his build and frame and have him weighed on a scale at a doctor's office. Well, it's apparent that, based on his height, he actually weighs too much. Next, someone built like him would go to the insurance company to be evaluated by what's called the Body Mass Index, or BMI, which is based on weight, height and surface area. It's obvious that after he is placed on one of these insurance chart tables, which incidentally are often used by many weight management studies and are possibly incorrectly, it is apparent that he is way "off the chart" and will not qualify for health or life insurance. Next, he comes to the ***Hot & Sexy Hormone Solution using my Youthful Blueprint System™***, where we perform a body composition analysis. This measures the actual components that make up weight. In other words, for the purposes of our discussion, the body is broken down into water weight, bone weight, fat weight and lean muscle mass weight. The most important two factors involve fat and muscle content. So, when looking at a person's body composition, the most important thing is to look at these two components.

In the case of someone like Arnold Schwarzenegger, you would find out that he is mostly muscle and has very little fat. So, in fact, body composition is more truly reflective of his weight situation and, therefore would be the most accurate way to assess someone at the initiation of a weight management program as they head toward long-term maintenance.

Interviewer: So, do you monitor muscle mass and fat mass, also known as body composition, throughout weight management and hormonal programs?

Dr. Moricz: That's right.

Interviewer: So what is it that the commercial programs are really afraid of?

Dr. Moricz: They are afraid that most of the initial weight loss is muscle. So while a person may initially weigh less, they are ultimately sacrificing metabolism because muscle burns calories, even when you sleep. This does not become evident until the weight loss hits a plateau and then patients start to gain weight again, since less muscle means less metabolism and calorie burning. So, unless steps are incorporated to preserve the lean muscle mass through specific approaches, such as nutritional measures and resistance training, the person may be worse off than before initiating the program.

So, in summary, as long as people are kept in the dark and invest in commercial programs that will drop weight without preserving muscle, they will never achieve long-lasting success.

Interviewer: So I've heard your clients say the *Hot & Sexy Hormone Solution using your Youthful Blueprint System ™* not only provides an initial body composition, but continual interval follow-up body composition monitoring that will demonstrate preservation and/or increase in muscle mass while showing continued fat loss.

Dr. Moricz: That is entirely correct.

Interviewer: Comment if you will on the experiences people have shared with you before implementing your Hormone Blueprint System.

Dr. Moricz: One of the large successes of my Hormone Blueprint System is the short amount of time in which it will end incorrect approaches that brought the person to the program in the first place. Put another way, there are four bothersome categories into which people have unwittingly been drawn:

> 1. **"Group meetings with disenchanted people."** Sitting with other people presumes that each individual has a group issue that can be solved with meetings that are not specific to one's metabolism and individualized needs. It is especially discouraging in a society that has the ability to dedicate resources "one-on-one" to achieve acceleration of goals in less time. Because really, that's what we're talking about—time. And in the process of aging, people don't realize that they are losing valuable time for achieving health and avoiding the pains of preventable disease. So, there is quite a bit of wasted time with people sitting in support-group-type formats, when, in fact, the problem is

much larger than talking it out, or listening to failed methods of reducing fat by simple changes in diet alone.

2. **"Prepared box meals."** There is a disturbing trend in committing people to the repetitive consumption of prepared boxed meals. This is a hyped marketing trend where, in fact, the actual ratio of carbohydrate and protein is not conducive to any success—even short-term success—at all. What it does drive is the need to purchase meals that tout calorie restriction without addressing the hormonal changes that the food composition of the meals encourages. These meals, found both in the supermarket and in advertised programs, need to be better scrutinized. It's unfortunate because by the growing trend of overweight and obese people in the United States, these companies can easily survive, even with a short-term trial of these products, by people suffering with these conditions.

3. **"Calorie counting frenzy."** This is an arduous approach, the value of which is even debated among experts. It's very difficult to reproduce even among experts what exact

calories, which are actually a unit of heat, for specific foods are among different studied protocols. The other issue is that calories—just like calculating weight mentioned earlier—presumes that the body is absent of hormones, and that the food composition in no way affects hormones. This is, once again, very flawed thinking. It will mislead people into thinking that calorie counting will give them long-term success, when actually the opposite is true. However, it is a big business and probably drives more people to the Hormone Blueprint System based on how discouraged they are with this kind of calorie-counting frenzy.

4.   **"Pill clinics."** These clinics use appetite-suppressants based on the idea that, if one can restrict appetite and increase metabolism for every client, that this alone will create long-lasting success. Without the structure of an individualized program and careful supervision, however, the use of pills assumes that everyone is similar in their long-term goals and preferences and will respond similarly, both short- and long-term. This approach is equally flawed and will generally be a revolving door of business that usually results in some modest

weight control and loss. But as soon as visits are discontinued and prescription weight loss medicines are discontinued, the person is often left helpless. Once again, this fourth category drives a number of clients to the Hormone Blueprint System, which evaluates clients based on their individualized short- and long-term goals, preferences, and realistic monitoring so that they can enter a maintenance phase where they ultimately require less monitoring with a supervising physician.

All in all, these four categories rarely address the metabolism issue and definitely ignore the hormonal one, which requires a deeper understanding and a particular individualization for each person.

Interviewer: Then I need to ask, what is the secret to the success of the *Hot & Sexy Hormone Solution using your Youthful Blueprint System ™?*

Dr. Moricz: Well, I do believe there are a number of qualified professional physician experts who are dedicated to weight management. I have simply taken a multi-layered approach that works together for increasing metabolism. Each program is broadly defined as Phase One and Phase Two.

Phase One, regardless of the individual program, is based on fat loss as an outcome. Phase Two is relapse prevention, or maintenance. In other words, once people have completed Phase One, they have achieved their ideal body fat percentage before they can enter Phase Two, which is maintenance of this newly achieved body composition. This is where things get confused in current approaches to weight management. It is only after the target body composition is reached, which is individualized to each client; that a client is allowed to go into the second phase, which is *maintenance*.

I think the reason why I did not involve myself in weight loss earlier in my clinical career is because I had to convince myself that there was a long-term approach to differentiate it from short-term failed approaches. And it was not until I had developed the Hormone Blueprint System that I could address both short- and long-term goals. Ultimately, the client is the outcome, and the body composition speaks for itself. In general, this program works far better for clients who are willing to dedicate themselves to long-lasting goals than for people who are accustomed to short-term success that ultimately leads to long-term failure.

Interviewer: For those people who are not familiar with your background and hormonal expertise, how would you describe how balancing hormones relates to weight control?

Dr. Moricz: I'm glad you asked that question. As you know, youth is perfect health, and when you are able to tune people's hormones back to their 20-year-old blueprint, weight management approaches take on a new level of success. That's why I really believe that it is futile in many cases to even take a multi-layered approach without first considering returning people to their 20-year-old hormonal blueprint. Because think about it again: When you're 20 and you need to lose fat, you certainly can cut back on calories and add some exercise with some incredible results. Taking advantage of that blueprint allows this system to achieve this more quickly, more pleasurably, and with more long-term success. Without understanding the hormonal aspects of weight management, I think a lot is being missed.

FREE GIFT!

Dr. Moricz has a FREE Weight Loss Special Report for you on the hormonal aspects of weight management and the secrets to true weight loss! Click below:

www.loseweightnow.solutions

Chapter 4: Sleep and Fatigue

Interviewer: Dr. Moricz, we often hear the terms "tired" and "fatigued." Are they really different, or are they the same thing?

Dr. Moricz: Think about this: When you're a small child or a baby and you get tired, you fall asleep without difficulty and get restful sleep that then allows you to be re-energized upon awakening. When adults get fatigued (for several reasons that I will explain later), they have the inability to get true rest and often have many interruptions in their sleep during the night. Therefore, they feel unrefreshed, as if they had never really gotten any rest at all. This is perhaps the most important aspect of understanding the difference between being tired and being fatigued.

Interviewer: Dr. Moricz, we often hear terms related to fatigue, including "fibromyalgia" and "chronic fatigue syndrome." Do these entities really exist?

Dr. Moricz: This is an issue that is still being debated among physicians. I can't tell you how many times physicians will say that there is no such thing as a fatigue-based disorder, such as fibromyalgia or chronic fatigue. I will often ask them, well, do they believe that there is something called migraines, true depression, irritable bowel syndrome and pelvic pain? They often will reply, "Well, yes, those are well-defined entities, but fibromyalgia and chronic fatigue don't really have any diagnostic features."

In other words, what they are telling me is that there's really no test because these conditions are diagnosed based on *exclusion*. Well, I can tell you of the above-mentioned problems, they are all diagnosed clinically. And even if one were to try to do diagnostic imaging for migraines and irritable bowel and pelvic pain, it would still be left to clinical criteria and validated pain questionnaires. It is unfortunate that for people who truly suffer from fatigue, be it fibromyalgia or chronic fatigue, that they are still being questioned.

Now, I'm not going to suggest that every person who complains of being fatigued has necessarily met the criteria for these conditions. What I am saying is that, in my work, I have created an approach that will treat the causation of fatigue, so it really shouldn't matter whether it meets the criteria for fibromyalgia or chronic fatigue syndrome, or some other explained reason for documented fatigue.

Interviewer: So, Dr. Moricz, what is the difference then between "chronic fatigue" and "fibromyalgia," and does it really matter?

Dr. Moricz: Well, it does matter from the methodology of medicine categorizing the condition so it can it be better studied, and so that studies can further break down subcategories that may not yet have been discovered. In other words, in the process of understanding a disorder, sometimes we figure out there's two or three, or more, variants that need to be analyzed differently and may have different treatments. So, in effect, it really does matter. Practically speaking, there is an overlap of two-thirds of the symptoms between the two entities. And for simplicity sake, many patients who are labeled with fibromyalgia do have some form of sleep disruption which affects their recovery and energy. Patients with chronic fatigue often have debilitating fatigue that may be related to poor adrenal and immune response.

In other words, they are different and can be categorized differently; however, many times there is quite an overlap of symptoms. So, I often believe that physicians often dismiss things that have not been comfortably diagnosed and where treatment is not necessarily causing immediate recovery.

Interviewer: So why doesn't treatment really work?

Dr. Moricz: Well, let me start by saying that when you break down fatigue disorders, oftentimes symptoms are treated with prescription medications and over-the-counter treatments. In the case of patients with fatigue disorders, oftentimes there is the abundant use of sedatives, sleep aids, antidepressants, stimulants and analgesics under the supervision of a physician. In other cases, over-the-counter approaches, including caffeine-based stimulants and over-the-counter analgesics and antihistamines are used by people looking for a *quick fix*.

Interviewer: Dr. Moricz, help us understand then what is the real basis of these fatigue disorders, and based on that, how does that affect treatment?

Dr. Moricz: That's an excellent question. Let me address a few different issues. Number one: Fatigue-related disorders may include abnormalities in proper sleep function, stress gland hormone production, and related problems including energy and inflammation. More specifically, these above issues must be evaluated correctly and approached very thoroughly. For instance, sleep is often treated with medications that do not allow for deep sleep.

Number two: Stress gland function is often overlooked with treatments including antidepressants and daytime stimulants. Also, energy function is rarely evaluated correctly with complete neglect of nutritional factors that really do make a big difference. Also in patients who also have inflammatory changes in the body, including the brain and the gut, without addressing these issues, patients are often in a fog and have difficulty with malabsorption. This further impairs day-to-day functioning and contributes to nutritional deficiencies.

Interviewer: Dr. Moricz, with chronic fatigue syndrome, is there a lot of talk about a possible viral connection?

Dr. Moricz: When evaluating the criteria of chronic fatigue syndrome, it appears there is some compromise in immune system. It is not entirely clear whether patients have sub-clinical infections, such as Lyme Disease that has been incompletely treated, or if there is also an underlying virus. But the bottom line is that there probably is some compromise in immune system that allows the infections to hover in the body without always producing better recognized infections that doctors are accustomed to treating.

Therefore, analysis of many protocols, such as those involved in attacking bacteria and viruses, will often involve long-term therapy. There are also some integrated approaches that suggest that the body must undergo a detoxification process, which will help the antibiotic and antiviral therapies work better.

So there really is a difference by criteria. However, since many people really don't get treated for these disorders, it's often better to see the whole picture of their fatigue, rather than get caught up in the fact that they may fit one category over the other. As I stated earlier, when you compare fibromyalgia and chronic fatigue patients, two thirds of the symptoms overlap. This makes it sometimes difficult to ignore that they may be variants of a similar disease process.

Interviewer: Dr. Moricz, since you are saying that there isn't a specific test for these illnesses, then what is the recommended approach for evaluating disruption in the patient's functioning?

Dr. Moricz: There are various ways to evaluate fatigue-related disorders. I will mention only a few because the details are beyond the scope of our conversation. Let me start by saying that there is a way to evaluate brain function through neurochemical testing, cellular function by doing intracellular nutrient analysis and hormonal testing to evaluate hormonal disruption. As a follow-up to your question, this then allows for balancing the brain chemicals through the use of nutrient balancing, including the use of intravenous therapy and proper hormonal balancing. The proper use of certain hormones produces an effect called *immunomodulation*, which means regulating the immune system. This is what you do not often hear as an approach. I can assure you that this has been the most valuable multi-layered approach for helping patients with fatigue that I have ever seen.

Interviewer: Having shared what you have about how fatigue affects people's day-to-day function, why do we commonly hear about weight gain in people suffering these problems?

Dr. Moricz: There are probably three key reasons to explain how sleep disruption affects weight gain. First, in normal patients who sleep well, such as young people, there is a natural rise in growth hormone at night followed by a rise in cortisol levels between 4 and 6 a.m. The growth hormone rise has several benefits, including repair of tissues and breakdown of fat. Cortisol, on the other hand, is a very critical hormone that is responsible for awakening in the 4-6 a.m. period. The problem with patients with sleep disruption is that they have inappropriate cortisol and adrenaline secretion, which disrupts their sleep cycle. Therefore, patients are deprived of the growth hormone benefit for lipolysis, or fat breakdown, along with tissue growth and recovery. Sleep doctors have identified in patients with disruptive sleep a condition of glucose intolerance the next day. In other words, patients' bodies have trouble handling their sugar the next day. This could easily be attributed to the inappropriate secretion of cortisol at night.

Let me also include a word or two about stress gland function. There are several critical hormones that are secreted. The ones of particular importance in this discussion include adrenaline, cortisol and DHEAS. Adrenaline is secreted throughout life and generally until the end of life. Cortisol secretion can be increased, especially under stress. There are conditions under chronic stress where there actually may be a decreased ability for the stress gland to secrete cortisol, even when the stress is resolved. This is called adrenal burnout. DHEAS is an extremely important hormone which is now being linked to immune protection, as well as the ability to deal with physical and emotional stress. It is not uncommon for patients with poor adrenal stress gland function to have a blunted cortisol response and very low DHEAS production. All of this is taking place in an individual who is sleeping poorly and who has poor daytime energy, which often leads to weight gain.

Interviewer: Dr. Moricz, how do patients with fatigue, such as fibromyalgia and chronic fatigue syndrome, present to you when seeking you out for weight control and not necessarily fatigue-related issues?

Dr. Moricz: A very critical approach to patients involves a complete evaluation of their day-to-day functioning. In addition to relevant hormonal and nutritional testing, it is very important to see the common thread between hormonal, nutritional and metabolic issues. Many times, the many people who are seeking me out for correction of their weight loss issues are in fact suffering with energy, sleep and hormonal issues. This is the very point of why I created the ***Hot & Sexy Hormone Solution using my Blueprint System***: to address the underlying issues for common conditions so that the root of the problem could be better attacked. And in the case of weight, correcting the underlying issues related to fatigue makes reaching a proper body composition far more likely and it will take a lot less time.

Interviewer: Based on the many people whom you see with fatigue, what is the most tragic thing that you often see?

Dr. Moricz: Many times, there are people who will never get the chance to be properly evaluated for their fatigue. I often feel bad because they are not treated well by the medical establishment. In other words, doctors treat symptoms without really understanding that this is a multi-layered issue. And when there is a multi-layered issue, it requires a multi-layered approach. Oftentimes, these patients will suffer not only from some of the problems that we discussed earlier, such as weight, but also develop immobility and ultimately disability. I have seen many patients on pain medications, sedatives and antidepressants, which have further compounded their energy issues and worsened their medical problems.

Interviewer: Dr. Moricz, what is the exact hormonal issue that you have identified and treated in fatigue-related disorders?

Dr. Moricz: Hormones are one of several issues in fatigue-related disorders. I feel that because the hormonal issues have been neglected to such a large degree that it possibly has the most valid justification for being addressed by the right hormonal specialist before other interventions are taken. Specifically, to answer your question, three general areas must be looked at carefully. First, the thyroid; then, the adrenal, or stress glands; and finally, the growth hormone axis. The details are beyond the scope of our discussion, but they do deserve further analysis. Even when these three hormonal systems are evaluated, oftentimes they are incorrectly interpreted by virtue of a blood test to be "abnormal"—even when the control center in the brain, the hypothalamus, is dysfunctional.

In other words, in medicine, there has been a great deal of attention paid to testing. The context of how the test is being used and whether it truly excludes a problem is far more important. To a clinically experienced hormonal specialist, however, the test is just a starting point. When looking at hypothalamic dysfunction, it often allows the specialist to see how the dysfunction of the control center is causing disruptive release signals to the thyroid, stress glands and growth hormone axis.

So, in summary, there are several hormonal factors for which the correct interpretation is lacking. This subsequently leaves the person thinking that they have been fully evaluated. But I can assure you that, in many cases, they have not. However, when they are properly evaluated and offered treatment possibilities, the results are like night and day.

Interviewer: Dr. Moricz, we often hear about insomnia or sleep-related disturbances. How do you define sleep disturbance so that you can better treat the person?

Dr. Moricz: Based on screening and interview, there are three important aspects of sleep that must be determined. The mistake that I have found over the years is that people are often asked, "How do you sleep?" Because they have become so accustomed to their poor quality of sleep over a long span of years, the answer is often less than satisfactory. What I would suggest is inquiring about sleep initiation, or the ability to get into good sleep, secondly the ability to stay asleep without interruptions or awakenings, and finally how restorative and refreshed the sleep is upon awakening. It is vital that these components be evaluated very carefully. Often the third question about restorative sleep can often clue one in to problems not only with sleep, but to patients suffering with undiagnosed pain disorders or nutritional deficiencies.

Interviewer: Then what do you do about the sleep problem once you have identified it?

Dr. Moricz: There is a systematic approach in the *Youthful Blueprint System™* that I have developed. First of all, the approach has to be individualized to the history and presentation of the person. A detailed review of sleeping habits, medical problems and use of medications is particularly noted. Next, weight issues can often compound sleep issues, such as sleep apnea. This is an important avenue that must be addressed. However, many do not have sleep apnea, but still suffer from very poor sleep. Based on a detailed functional medicine questionnaire review, the issues mentioned above, including initiation, interruption and non-restorative sleep, are diagnosed. Then, based on hormonal, neurochemical and nutritional testing, deficiencies to confirm clinical suspicion is pursued.

If the person has a defined sleep problem based on this detailed review, I use a proven system for building each client an individualized sleep supplement to replenish restful sleep. This has been an extremely successful individualized approach for helping people regain restful sleep.

Interviewer: Dr. Moricz, the more I talk with you, the more I feel that what we are calling medical problems may not really be medical problems at all. Am I taking too much of a leap in saying that?

Dr. Moricz: That's right. Once the neurochemicals of the brain and hormones of the body are balanced correctly, you are no longer in *imbalance*. It would be much better to attack the hormonal imbalance than give a person a premature diagnosis. I cannot tell you how many people I have treated who were once incorrectly labeled as fat, depressed, lazy or poorly disciplined. Unfortunately, they were often flooded with prescription medications by medical practitioners, when in some of these cases it furthered addictions and weight gain problems.

Interviewer: Dr. Moricz, thank you for your eye-opening insight into how you are helping people get restful sleep and youthful energy through your *Hot & Sexy Hormone Solution using your Youthful Blueprint System™.*

FREE GIFT! Dr. Moricz has a FREE Sleep Quiz for you to take that will give you custom results! Discover how to go from sleep deprived to Sleeping Beauty! To claim your free gift, go to: www.mybodyhormone.com

Chapter 5: Youth is Beauty

[Skin]

Interviewer: Dr. Moricz, everywhere we turn there is some new procedure or some never before mentioned therapy for beautiful skin. Are we missing something or has our understanding of the skin dramatically changes?

Dr. Moricz: The biggest and heaviest organ in your body – skin is in a constant state of flux. It divides, repairs itself, removes old pieces of itself and mounts a response to constant changes within and outside your body. Skin not only protects our internal organs including bone and soft tissue from the external environment but also packages our body into different compartments.

A FEW SIMPLE WORDS ABOUT ANATOMY. There are cells called *fibroblasts* which create support fibres known as connective tissue, specifically collagen and elastin. Collagen is responsible for firmness and elastin gives skin its stretchiness. There is an outer layer known as the epidermis which protects the deeper layer known as the dermis where the fibroblasts make the collagen and elastin mentioned above. Within the dermis are also hair follicles, sweat and sebaceous glands which produce sweat and oily sebum, respectively. Beneath the dermis is a primarily fatty layer called subcutaneous tissue which helps insulate heat and cushion the body.

What is often forgotten is that two thirds of your skin is filled with water and the remaining third is mostly protein and some and even less fats.

Interviewer: So why is it Dr. Moricz that there is so much focus on the outer layer for keeping women beautiful?

Dr. Moricz: Your skin has a built in repair and renewal system that makes sure that fresh skin cells make their way to the surface while ridding your body of old skin cells. The structural cells are constantly active keeping the skin resilient, fresh and intact. Think of your skin layers as a complex factory that is constantly renewing the appearance of your beautiful skin.

Interviewer: Then why is it that as we age that our skin seems to age with us?

Dr. Moricz: A lot could be said about chronological age and the way that aging is measured in the body. There are two basic causes of aging that can be divided into two groups: 1) Genetic Factors; and 2) Random Events.

Genetic factors of aging focus on how genes program lifecycles of cells and the death of cells as well. Random events focus on how cells deal with wear and tear, waste removal, recovery against free radicals and the cells' energy powerhouses, the way that cells deal with sugar, poor immune systems and hormonal effects. Most clients that I see could be evaluated for all of these causes but more practically after obvious metabolic issues which cause inflammation are dealt with, we usually have to tackle the effects of hormonal imbalance and cell protection against free radicals and environmental toxins. Interestingly, hormones can modulate the immune system and also have antioxidant activity as well.

On a more practical level aging is often characterized by changes in physical appearance especially skin, hair, muscle, bones and fat tissue which corresponds to what would be expected in a person of the same chronological age. With regards to the skin, it may show wrinkling, thinning and swelling under the eyes. One of the main reasons why clients will seek me out is to tackle premature aging or what they call *"aging before their years"*

Interviewer: Dr. Moricz, women who are reading this are often bombarded with the media on all types of beauty issues. Many of these are often linked with a "magic wand" type cure for everything from wrinkling to thinning skin and loss of firmness particularly of the face. If these therapies were really the "cure all" then why does it seem like more and more women are running to the cosmetic counter and the cosmetic surgeon?

Dr. Moricz: The real question is *"Are women aging before their years?"* Oftentimes therapies are being recommended <u>without</u> a basic individualized evaluation of a woman's beauty in the first place. In other words, when I see clients, a detailed 3D skin analysis, skin quiz and hormonal evaluation precede any discussion of therapy.

In other words, when looking at the most obvious issues in aging skin, I often break down the issues into damage to the skin itself, underlying layers and structural support including muscle and fat that give skin its proper support. Put differently, you would never think of doing landscaping and decorating around your house without properly building the foundation and structures like walls and roof.

It is true that much of what fills the media for "problem skin" involves discussion of acne, sun damage, which we call photo-aging, and ways of helping the turnover of the skin so that the top layer sheds itself quicker and hides any sign that the skin is sloughing slowly as women get chronologically older.

Interviewer: Dr. Moricz you mentioned something interesting – 3D computerized skin analysis. What more can you share with us on the benefits of this?

Dr. Moricz: You are correct. The basis of what I do for my clients is return people back to their youthful blueprint. In other words, in an earlier chapter you had read about how youth is perfect health. Well it is true that at an earlier point in life most women had perhaps the most "perfect combination" of natural chemicals and hormones in their body. Not coincidentally they also had the most beautiful skin that they would ever have in their life. So while I am not certainly against approaches for protecting the skin, increasing antioxidants to protect against free radicals and regimens including anti-inflammatory diets, what I have found is that the evaluation was highly inadequate. In other words, in advanced science it is necessary to utilize the most advanced techniques to identify the issues at hand.

Using 3D computerized analysis, I am able to uncover problems that lurk beneath the top layer of the skin and subsequently can design a custom protocol which addresses these exact issues. This avoids any guessing or trial and error which most women reading this are well conditioned to avoid. In my upcoming book: *Are You Suffering From The Invisible Woman Syndrome*, I will detail more about this unique technology that is giving women an unfair advantage for youthful skin even when nothing had previously worked.

Like my youthful blueprint system, brain blueprint system, knowing our skin blueprint changes everything as far as receiving results and the speed in which you can reach these outcomes.

Interviewer: For those women who are not immediately able to access you in one of your VIP programs and undergo a skin blueprint, what other suggestions can you offer?

Dr. Moricz: To help women who know deep in their heart that having their skin blueprint gives them the simple certainty of going from where they are now to youthfully glowing skin, I have prepared some very valuable strategies that could be started in the comfort of their own home. What I will do at the end of our discussion is be sure that each and every reader has access to my *Skin and Beauty Quiz* as well as an opportunity to get a "sneak peek" of what happens for VIP clients at Body Hormone Balance Anti-aging Center.

Specifically, there are methods which I design that are very different yet have proven effective and safe solutions which women love for beautiful skin. One aspect of what I do that may be different is not only addressing nutritional components which are a significant but not the only contributor to their skin's beauty. To better evaluate hormonal effects, I have devised methods for assessing skin thickness, elasticity, hydration, underlying muscle tone and wrinkling.

Because of my background in designing hormonal blueprints for my VIP clients, I have expanded into designing skin blueprints which also address the hormonal factors that are often neglected in the flurry of Madison Avenue style interventions and aggressive cosmetic procedures. We look at this as not only giving women skin that is radiant but also not forgetting to rebuild the quality of the underlying skin layers and its cell rejuvenation to make the skin both firm and elastic. But none of this happens without an *individualized skin blueprint.*

Interviewer: Is it true, Dr. Moricz that you have designed not only a skin miracle system but also Dr. Moricz' ultimate sleep solution™ for delivering "over the top" beauty results using deep restful sleep?

Dr. Moricz: Well it is true that beauty sleep has critical effects on beautiful skin. There is one confession I have that often astounds my VIP clients: Of all the problems that I could overcome with the use of natural hormonal therapies, the one that <u>I could not overcome with hormonal therapy alone</u> is achieving deep refreshing sleep for clients who could not get the youthful beauty sleep they needed. As a result, I developed a complete system – not a *'try this bottle and hope it works approach'* – that restores the six natural sleep chemicals that are missing in over ninety percent of sleep sufferers. Using this approach, within two months my clients wake up fully refreshed ready to take on the day without any noticeable fatigue throughout the afternoon, forego stimulants or five hour energy drinks to keep them alert, experience enjoyable evenings and start the cycle over by falling asleep, staying asleep and waking up feeling younger each day.

Interviewer: This is very different. What originally inspired you to create this "one off" system and what is your mission for women's beauty?

Dr. Moricz: A word or two about my Skin Miracle System™. After befriending a pioneer in skin UV analysis, I was inspired to design individualized systems very different than what women were experiencing in the dermatologic and cosmeceutical world; the basic difference being in developing a woman's skin blueprint first and then designing a pharmaceutical grade solution based on her skin type. I have even guaranteed taking "10 years off their face in less than 10 days" with my **Exclusive European Rejuvenation System**. I have now released my over the counter **Skin Miracle System™** without a prescription to the general public because I have no conceivable way of helping so many women who have written to me and essentially twisted my arm to make this available to them.

[Hair]

Interviewer: Dr. Moricz, there are hundreds if not thousands of hair products to keep women beautiful. Do you believe we have a hair fascination epidemic?

Dr. Moricz: Wherever you turn, you are reminded how to regain the body, bounce and gloss of your hair. It is difficult to cover the topic of beauty without discussing something very fundamental to your self-image and billboard to the world about who you are – your hair. In the Unites States fifty billion dollars a year is spent on hair. On the surface it might sound like expenditures on shampoos and colouring when, in fact, the laundry list of hair care products seems to be growing every day. From glazing to repair products and touch up agents the list goes on even though the biology of your hair follows the same principles.

Interviewer: What are the fundamental basics about hair that women really need to know?

Dr. Moricz: The essentials of your hair revolve around hair follicles and for the purposes of our discussion on beautiful hair it will focus on the hair on your head. A little bit later you'll have the opportunity to discover essential signs of imbalance in your body based on the health of your hair – hormones and nutrition. The hair follicle starts deep below the skin with the hair shaft most recognizable to you. The hair shaft is composed of a protein we recognise as keratin with an inner and outer layer making up most of the hair shaft.

Interviewer: What problem areas do you often help women with?

Dr. Moricz: A lot of discussions that women begin asking as they chronologically age revolve around thinning, dryness, brittleness, comb-ability, loss of hair color which turns up as grey and white hair and just as importantly is hair loss. A lot of space could be dedicated to the biology of hair loss whether it occurs as male pattern baldness, diffuseness (all over hair loss), or patches. For the sake of our discussion we will skip infections and serious diseases which can affect the turnover and growth of hair.

Having mentioned hair loss, it can take two to three years for the growth phase of hair to be complete with much shorter time for resting and "falling out" phases as well. In other words, even though the hair that you see is made up of keratin which is dead, the follicle below the scalp is very active in trying to renew the hair and take you through different cycles.

Interviewer: What about the role of hormones on women's health and hair?

Dr. Moricz: Briefly stated, hormonal changes including an imbalance between female and male hormones as well as the stronger conversion of the male hormone to a more powerful form which is very typical also in men, can account for loss and turnover of hair. Other hormones including those involved with stress and the thermostat gland we call the thyroid can affect the quality as well as patterns of hair loss.

Oftentimes evaluation of hair is based on thickness, hair volume, hair loss, whether at the top of the head or diffuse (all over), as well as brittleness and dryness; changes in hair color are based on the biology of well-known hormones which actually give you natural hair color and are known to "drop off" with chronological age.

Interviewer: Dr. Moricz, couldn't women just take mega doses of B Vitamins or the "so called" hair vitamin supplements?

Dr. Moricz: So while no-one is against use of vitamins and hoping the correction of one hormone or two, and use of modern hair products and treatments, it often makes sense to evaluate the report card of your hair's health and not only uncover proven ways to transform the beauty of your hair but also restore any health imbalances that gave you this problem with your hair in the first place. To help you with this, please refer to the **beauty quiz** on how you can transform the health of your beauty and keep you healthy too.

[Nails]

Interviewer: Dr. Moricz, everywhere women turn there is a lot of focus on their nails. What critical information are we missing about the nails as a sign of beauty?

Dr. Moricz: A part of the body that gets quite a bit of attention is your nails. For example, women spend a good deal of effort to show off their nails with manicures and pedicures. Not only are your nails a sign of beauty but they can also uncover hidden deficiencies in your body. These deficiencies can be in the form of hormonal and nutritional imbalances that surface as abnormalities in your nails.

Something that is commonly forgotten is that your nails can grow about a tenth of a millimetre a day which translates into a fingernail taking about six months to fully grow out. So, when you remove the polish and cover up of your nails what we're really looking at it not just the beauty of your nails but the health of your nails which can uncover problems with your health.

Interviewer: What tell-tale signs should alert women about their nail health?

Dr. Moricz: The anatomy of the nail most visible to you is the nail plate which is locked into the skin along the nail fault to keep it in place. The nail bed which lies beneath the skin is critical for producing the actual fingernail or toenail plate.

There isn't enough room here to completely cover infections like fungus or other skin conditions and injuries to nails. However there are some tell-tale signs about your nail and internal health. Particular areas of concern on the nail are splitting and brittleness, white spots, greyish borders, and spoon shaped nails. Below you will have an opportunity to take a *beauty quiz* that will help you discover more than you ever could imagine about your health and beauty, through analysis of your nails.

Take Dr. Moricz' Beauty Quiz and receive your custom skin blueprint results! www.skinblueprint.com

CHAPTER 6: SECRET OF SUCCESS

Interviewer: Dr. Moricz, we've heard so much about the transformations that people have undergone with the Body Hormone Balance System. But before we talk about that, though, we often hear about how dysfunctional medicine has become. What are your thoughts about this?

Dr. Moricz: You know, a lot has been said about success with modern medicine in the twenty-first century. This is particularly true for people suffering coronary events and receiving end-of-life care. What is truly remarkable is how far we've come in emergency room interventions and critical care units to perform heroic efforts for saving people's lives. The question arises, what about everyday help and particularly preventative help that would lessen the reliance on the critical care and emergency room interventions? Now, that's when it gets a little bit interesting. See, over the last ten years, I have started to track my patients' weight and medications. In other words, when they returned for their yearly visits, I started to notice a trend: Their weights were increasing and their reliance on prescription medications was growing. It seemed to me that for as many doctor and hospital visits as there are each year that reliance on pharmaceutical care would decline. In fact, quite the opposite was true.

The list of medications, imaging studies, and required follow-up appointments was growing in my private practice population. One might argue that my patients were aging and therefore it would be expected that they'd have increased intervention. Well, I started to look at their weight, which started to trouble me at first because they were suffering ten, twenty, and thirty-plus pounds of weight gain. I could not entirely exclude that some of the medications, which were known to be associated with weight gain, were contributing, in part, to the problem. I also started to notice decrease in energy as a major issue after the initiation of these medications, along with the growing weight issue.

It would be very convenient to blame everything on inactivity and the illness itself. And I can't entirely exclude that behavioral patterns do not contribute to the problem. But what about these medications, and what about this documented change in weight?

Interviewer: Well, Dr. Moricz, what did you do to investigate this issue?

Dr. Moricz: After traveling all over the country and meeting with different physicians who had some level of success in treating weight, fatigue and hormonal issues, I started to see a pattern. I also plowed through mounds and mounds of scientific research papers and spent thousands of hours sorting out things that did and did not make sense to me. I didn't disagree about the *effort* that was being made by clinicians, researchers, pharmaceutical companies and hospital-based agencies. What I didn't understand was why the whole process was so dysfunctional.

In other words, what common thread would explain why patients had to see so many doctors, even after they saw their primary care physician to sort out what was appearing to me as a recurrent problem? As mentioned in our earlier discussions, I started to correlate not their chronological age, but the inflammation and hormonal changes in their body as setting them up for the medical treatments and medications that were required based on our current practice in conventional medicine.

And I started to question whether what we were calling a successful outcome was really successful at all.

How can you tell patients that theirs was a successful outcome when they have gained an enormous amount of weight and have to rely on multiple medications and still can't be as fit or enjoy life as they used to? I felt I had to do better than that.

Interviewer: So, Dr. Moricz, before you tell us more about how you designed the model of your Hormone Blueprint System, tell us what impact you think dysfunctional medicine has on the day-to-day economics of Americans, as well as their psychological well-being?

Dr. Moricz: First, I do not claim to have an economic study on what I am about to say. And you might even call it an educated guess or future observation. I'm not afraid to commit to what I am about to say, but I would like to propose it as a discussion for further thought by people who truly are trained in economics.

Imagine this…

> The very people who are suffering from weight-related issues are able to be managed one-on-one with marked success so that they no longer have to rely on "eating out" and "eating an abundance of unhealthy food." Also, imagine that they no longer have the heavy reliance on the big pharmaceutical industry medications,

which of course may mean that they don't require as many doctor visits, nor do they have possible side effects that require further pharmacologic interventions. And, in particular, I am describing a drop-in incidence of what is now known as *metabolic syndrome*, which includes components such as obesity, diabetes, lipid disorders and high blood pressure. Therefore, what I am suggesting is a change.

I would suggest a different approach to people's health by ridding them of their need for dependency on unhealthy food, particularly that of the restaurant industry, and less reliance on multiple pharmaceutical medications. But would it kill the American economy (which depends so heavily on the food and pharmaceutical industries)?

You asked about the psychological well-being of people. One of the trends that I noticed at the initiation of my Hormone Blueprint System is the need to establish an **individualized** protocol that attacks the problematic role of food as stimulation, when it should serve as a method of reasonable satisfaction. I won't go into details on how the brain chemistry is affected by over-indulgence with the wrong types of food, but I will say that one of the successful outcomes I see consistently in weight management clients is the realization that food is now satisfying to them, and no longer a compelling stimulatory necessity.

Another factor that is also at the forefront of these programs is defining the roles of improper eating habits associated with eating out as being the center of social activity. Put differently, food can be seen as a survival mechanism, but in excess, it does become a substitute or an excuse of social activity, which is extremely unhealthy for peoples' well-being. And why is that? Despite the negative consequences, the overreliance on food as stimulation gets in the way of staying healthy.

Interviewer: Well Dr. Moricz, that's a very bold look at how the future of weight management medicine will ultimately succeed with people who are suffering from being overweight and obese. But tell me, how does a hormonal specialist get involved with weight management in the first place?

Dr. Moricz: I'm really glad you asked that. Years ago, I would have never imagined that I would be as involved as I am now in helping people with their weight problems. I never really believed the approach we had in place is really a system at all. And, as we discussed earlier, it is more likely to lead to disappointment because it was a "hands-off approach" that even made clinicians uncomfortable.

So, to answer your question, adipose, or fat tissue (particularly the deep fat tissue we call visceral fat), is the largest hormonal organ in the body. This comes as such a shock to most people! They don't realize the number of important, and possibly damaging, hormones and chemicals that are secreted from fat tissue. This includes female hormone, corticosteroids, and inflammatory chemicals called *cytokines*, and even chemicals that trigger the kidney to increase blood pressure above normal. Inflammation affects hormones as do hormones affect inflammation. There are even scientific models looking at how these inflammatory chemicals in the body can affect the control center of the brain.

Clients who have successfully transformed not only their way of thinking but their body composition and their overall future health have often asked me why would a doctor who comes from a hormonal background get involved with weight management. Well, it is very apparent that there is a lot more involvement of hormones with fat storage and inflammation than is currently seen on television, the internet and in print media.

Interviewer: Dr. Moricz that is fascinating information. What about some specific examples of diseases in men and women? Would you comment on some examples that might help us understand what, in fact, is really going on?

Dr. Moricz: I would be glad to. First, let's talk about diabetes in men; an area that I feel has suffered unnecessary neglect. There is enough information in scientific literature and the clinical studies that diabetes is very reversible in men. Let me first start by saying that when I do hormonal testing in men, particularly when we are talking about Type 2 diabetes, which is diabetes developed later in life, what is apparent is that there is an inverse relationship between insulin levels and male hormone.

Newer studies are showing that there is an inflammatory effect on the testes, which is where male hormone production takes place, by high insulin levels. Also, male hormone can sensitize the body to insulin, therefore making it work better. So, when patients gain fat, especially noticeable in diabetes, the fat actually produces more estrogen, which then binds up the male hormone making things even worse. So, there is this vicious cycle where men are not only making less male hormone and having less available, but they are also being affected by estrogen, which is a female hormone, as it floods their system. This, by the way, is critical, because high estrogen levels are associated with thickening of the blood vessels with cholesterol.

Now, let's talk about an example in women. In order to understand in simple terms what systems are affected by estrogen, it is important to see at what levels in the body estrogen works. Estrogen affects the brain, the breasts and the uterus, and is produced by visceral fat.

Why is this important? Well, in early female sexual development, the breasts are far more sensitive than the uterus to estrogen. That's why girls will normally develop breasts as the first part of sexual maturation. A growing problem is early development of breasts sometimes even before eight years of age. In women in their 20's to 40's, excessive estrogen production, particularly from visceral fat, causes everything from anxiety and pregnancy-like symptoms, including bloated-ness, breast tenderness and fluid retention. In other women, because of the excessive amount of female hormone, they have abnormal uterine bleeding. As a function of decreased metabolism and increased fat gain, there is even more estrogen produced than in their earlier years. So, in both men and women, there are some specific examples of processes that are affecting what we are treating as medical conditions.

Interviewer: Dr. Moricz, comment if you will on how environmental toxicities may be contributing to this problem even further.

Dr. Moricz: That is an excellent point. If we look at exposure to plastics and other chemicals foreign to the body in our everyday environment, there are what is called *xenoestrogens*, which means they look and behave like estrogens, though they aren't the exact molecule. What does this have to do with men and women? For one, in men, we have seen a huge decline in testosterone male hormone levels, as well as sperm counts. In women, we have seen measurable increases in hormone carriers that are related to increased estrogen in the body. This may cause all the hazards of excessive estrogen in women's bodies, including female cancers.

Interviewer: Dr. Moricz, tell us then, are there ways to measure these effects indirectly?

Dr. Moricz: As one part of the *Body Hormone Balance System* evaluation, we measure both in men and women the male and female hormones present, along with a carrier molecule called sex hormone binding globulin. Simply stated, the carrier molecule may be a hormone itself. So, there are ways to measure some inappropriate elevations or decreases, depending on the individual.

Interviewer: How does that influence treatment?

Dr. Moricz: When the abnormality can be correlated with symptoms, then an individualized hormone therapy program can be tailored to alter this carrier molecule's level, and ultimately make clinical differences in the patient's well-being, body composition, and other measureable health parameters.

Interviewer: Dr. Moricz, let's talk about hormonal testing. With all the technology available for laboratory testing, are we doing a better job for people?

Dr. Moricz: There is an important point to be made about laboratory testing, especially when and how to test, as well as how to use the test. In the beginning of medical training, student doctors are often taught that we don't treat tests, we treat people. With the abundance of requirements and demands made on something palpable such as a lab test, a lot has been lost in the interaction between the doctor and the patient. What is far more critical is the clinical experience and deeper understanding by the physician of what is the expected outcome of a test before it is done. I think it has always been said best in medical training that "You order a test in order to answer a specific question." So, in order to gain a better appreciation for why a test is ordered in a specific setting, there needs to be clinical experience to guide the use of the test and the limits of what the test will tell you.

Interviewer: Do you think there is an overreliance on laboratory testing?

Dr. Moricz: As a general statement, I believe that there are cases when there is such an abundance of testing done because there is not a strong enough relationship between the physician and the person being treated.

Therefore, it is more important to develop as good an interview with a person and to have the person disclose as much of what is really going on with his or her health. And I do believe that there are times when there is an overreliance on laboratory tests as a substitute for sorting out what is really going on with the person.

I am privileged to be able to choose the people with whom I work because I find that there is a commitment from the person being treated to be an active participant. So, in my own practice, I don't find an overreliance on laboratory studies, but I do find myself explaining to people what the pitfalls are of too much testing, and whether the tests would even help us change our course of therapy. That's why hormonal balancing is such an important science, as well as an art.

Interviewer: Dr. Moricz, comment on some of the art and what your expertise could tell our readers about what to expect.

Dr. Moricz: Well, earlier we talked about a dysfunctional model of medicine that often relies on several different referrals to figure out possibly one or two underlying causes. This is not to suggest that people do not need to see different specialists when recommended, but it does suggest that trying to identify hormonal deficiencies as correlated to signs and symptoms of illness may, in fact, have a larger role than we once thought. Put differently, some medical problems that we're calling medical problems may be, in part, *hormonal imbalances.*

So, as an important follow-up to the earlier question, it is important to use laboratory testing carefully, once an adequate evaluation of specific issues in a person has been done. The timing, modality, and the appropriateness of a lab test are critical factors when ordering the test in the first place.

Think of hormonal expertise and hormonal balancing as a well-thought-out chess game. With every manipulation of one or two hormones, there may be effects both positive and negative on others. I think one of the biggest problems is the idea that people would have one or two hormones checked later in life and adjust those hormones in *isolation*. I'll talk more about this later, but just so you know, there is a huge nosedive in hormones as early as the late 20's and early 30's in men and women.

Interviewer: Dr. Moricz, give us some examples of why people are currently seeing doctors for hormonal issues, and what that may mean for their improvement.

Dr. Moricz: Well, let's start with a few examples. Many women will seek out an OBGYN doctor for female hormonal deficiencies in their 40's and 50's. Men will often see out an UROLOGIST for male hormonal deficiency symptoms. Diabetics may seek out a MEDICAL ENDOCRINOLOGIST because their diabetes is becoming more brittle and hard to manage. Still others will see FAMILY DOCTORS for day-to-day fatigue and energy hormone issues. As stated earlier, there is a huge nosedive in hormones as early as the late 20's or early 30's, depending on the individual. I think a big fault in the way that hormone evaluation and treatment is being handled is that people are making it too late to the doctor, and this means that they are already in trouble.

If I were to withhold treatment for already symptomatic people because their hormonal laboratory tests were in the "normal" range (based on population values for ages 5-80), then I would deny over half the people I see effective medical therapy that would soon relieve their symptoms and improve their quality of life. That leaves a lot to be desired.

In addition, many of the people that I see who may not have any symptoms at all are already showing early signs of deficiency in multiple hormones. So, to use the example above, if different patients (both men and women) saw different doctors, they may have only one or two hormones tuned. What that implies is that only one or two hormones are explaining a number of changes in their body.

Interviewer: Dr. Moricz, this is fascinating information on our current perspective of medicine. I cannot imagine that your model of the Hormone Blueprint System would not have application to many people who are still looking for relief. What can you tell us about the critical elements of your Hormone

Blueprint System that have enabled so many people to enjoy success?

Dr. Moricz: Well, let me start by stating that when I say an *"Individualized Approach,"* I really do mean that. This involves a detailed functional medicine approach with a questionnaire and an interview that really focuses on improving the clinical outcome of the client. Now this seems obvious and many might say, "Well, that's why people become physicians." However, what has happened with the role of insurance companies and what I call a clipboard-type system is that the physician is often burdened with so many checklists and computerized record requirements that sometimes it's a chase to the paperwork, which leaves time not well spent. So after an adequate assessment of a functional questionnaire, there needs to be correlation between signs and symptoms, including validation of these abnormalities. Then there is a careful analysis of appropriately relevant tests so that a treatment plan with options can be created for the well-being and functional health of the client. Ultimately, the safe use of hormonal balancing can often alleviate anxiety and give a structured plan for success.

Interviewer: Then how does the one-step model of current medicine really address reaching successful outcomes with clients?

Dr. Moricz: I don't really think it can. In constructing programs, I carefully designed the ability to have multiple individualized one-on-one visits so that fine-tuning of interventions could be monitored and adjusted earlier, rather than later. In other words, the therapy has to be in harmony with unintended hormonal changes that can occur. That's really why I consider the Hormone Blueprint System to be a functional approach to hormones and wellness.

Interviewer: Dr. Moricz, this discussion has certainly created a new vision for what you are describing as a functional approach. Comment, if you will, on future directions that you predict with regard to hormones and nutrition.

Dr. Moricz: In the field of hormones, I believe there will be even further discoveries about the roles played by hormones and inflammation. In other words, we know through the field of *immunomodulation* that there is a greater correlation on how hormones and inflammation regulate each other. Another important area is hormones as *neurosteroids* on brain function.

Others include the protective effect of hormones on Alzheimer's and other neurodegenerative diseases.

Still, there is some exciting information on the effect of hormones on the heart, as well. Studies are correlating the effect of growth hormone and male hormone on heart function. We know now that male hormone can dilate coronary blood vessels and help the pumping action of the heart. Receptors are also being found with growth hormone as well. Possibly the future may involve the use of cardiac stents with male hormone to prevent further thickening of coronary wall plaques.

There is still another area regarding autoimmune disorders in women, because as they get older, they have a decrease in male hormone production. Male hormones can regulate the immune system, and in women, this is an extremely important area, especially in regard to rheumatoid arthritis and lupus.

Finally, an interesting area would be the effect of hormones on inflammatory bowel diseases, such as Crohn's disease and Ulcerative Colitis. There is a study on growth hormone and a possible healing effect to improve quality of bowel function in Crohn's patients. I would like to see further studies done on the re-healing of the gut lining with the use of growth hormone and growth factor agents so that patients who suffer greatly from this disorder would have a better quality of life. Equally as exciting is the potential of stem cell therapy for rejuvenating hormonal glandular function.

With regard to nutrition, I would like to see the implementation of more aggressive nutritional factors as a way to prevent disease. This would require further identification of early nutritional deficiencies. There is growing data that associates nutritional deficiencies with specific medical disorders. Once an integrated approach can be started with the use of nutraceutical supplementation, along with herbal replacements, we may see its greater role in preventative medicine.

With regard to the brain and muscle energy, it is now known that certain supplements will protect energy production. Here, too, it would be nice to see how earlier intervention might also protect the brain and muscle function, since energy is a huge issue as we get older.

Lastly, I would like to see an expansion of what is called neurochemical testing, where brain chemicals are tested so there will be less reliance on psychotropic medications and more specific balancing of brain hormonal chemicals so that people can lead more productive lives without the side effects that many antidepressants and stimulants cause.

Interviewer: Dr. Moricz, thank you once again for your insights on the Hormone Blueprint System and what the future of your program may provide.

CHAPTER 7: THE REASON FOR THE HORMONE BLUEPRINT SYSTEM

Earlier, a very critical promise was made to you. The purpose of writing this book, the *Hot & Sexy Hormone Solution* was to avoid trial/error and all the pain, suffering and loss of quality of life that goes with that kind of approach. It might seem that wellness in the United States is already within easy reach. However, doctors' offices and clinics throughout the United States would demonstrate otherwise. People suffering with energy, focus and metabolic issues have filled multiple appointment slots all with the disappointment of increased pill taking, expensive testing and continued poor health.

The concept that *"Youth Is Perfect Health"* is perhaps the most critical chapter for you to understand in this book. In other words, when you are returned to your 20-year-old *"blueprint,"* you return to possibly the best hormonal and cellular function that you have ever had. That's why youth is perfect health.

A lesson that was made clear throughout medical school was that, first, one had to have an understanding of "normal" before studying disease. Why is this relevant? Because these days, people as early as their late 20's are aging well before their years. Without reiterating the exact causes of aging as described in earlier chapters, the fact that it is happening in younger and younger people should set off alarms. I am not here to state that aging is reversible, and I do not necessarily believe it is, but theoretically, aging should be able to be slowed.

So, you may be wondering, who was the individual mentioned at the beginning of this book who was so critical to compel me to create the ***Youthful Blueprint System*** ™? Who suffered so chronically with issues including sleep, fatigue and immune dysfunction? Whose suffering do I credit for taking another look and possibly an unexplored approach to healing the body?

The ANSWER is ME.

I was this individual. I was the medical-doctor-turned-patient who could not benefit from the very system that trained me, despite multiple specialty doctor visits, workups and treatment plans. Despite all of this effort, I was left without any significant improvement. I did, however, come across a few select physicians, who because of their personal health and that of their families also took another look at approaches outside the usual prescription-writing protocol. And while I did have some early improvement as a patient under their medical care, what I really learned from them was that I had to become a student again. They got me started, but what eventually made the difference was becoming a student who had to figure out the reason for the approach that was safe, effective and reproducible, and that's what made all the difference.

Earlier, I described how **Youth Is Perfect Health**, and how taking a look at the *blueprint* that kept you healthy at 20 is possibly one of the biggest keys to keeping you from getting unhealthy in the first place. I will freely admit that the development of the Hormone Blueprint System greatly benefitted me.

What really has been rewarding to me is what it has done for the many patients who came to me also with previously poor results, despite multiple doctor visits, workups, prescription medicines and continued poor health. Once they applied the systems that I have briefly described in this book, now known as the **Youthful Blueprint System ™**, they, too, were tapping into their 20-year-old blueprint with a reduced reliance on prescription medications, fewer doctors' visits, and avoidance of the disability and pain, which was clearly in their near future. It is to my patients that I credit the development of this program. It is because of my personal suffering and necessity to find a better approach that I set out to start what is likely an evolution of treatment for people.

It is with great appreciation that I thank all of the doctors and patients who made me rethink everything I ever learned and taught me the importance of becoming a student again.

In closing, I urge you to remember that the body has an ability to heal itself. It will do this in many different ways. It's our obligation to see how we can promote this healing as we head well into the twenty-first century.

It is likely that every healing art has something to offer for each condition. It is also likely that one healing art does it better than the other for each specific condition, but at times multiple approaches may be extremely helpful.

Thank you for your participation in reading this book and for your interest in the *Hot & Sexy Hormone Solution* and my custom designed *Blueprint System.*

FREE GIFTS TO HELP YOU!

- **Take Dr. Moricz' Beauty Quiz and receive your custom skin blueprint results!** www.skinblueprint.com

- **Take Dr. Moricz' Sleep Quiz and Discover *How to go from Sleep Deprived to* Sleeping Beauty:** www.mybodyhormone.com
- **Discover New Secrets to Weight Loss:** www.loseweightnow.solutions

TO SHARE YOUR LIFE CHANGING SUCCESS STORY BECAUSE OF THIS "OVER THE TOP YOUTHFUL BLUEPRINT SYSTEM" PLEASE FORWARD YOUR CONTACT INFORMATION TO:

CONTACT INFORMATION

George F. Moricz, M.D.,

Founder, Hormonal Blueprint System

Telephone: 561-240-4900

http://www.bodyhormonebalance.com/

For the latest schedule of Live Events near you, go to:

www.doctormoricz.com

ABOUT THE AUTHOR

As a thought leader in anti-aging, Dr. Moricz has integrated hormonal balancing, weight management and control over fatigue. He has advanced cutting edge anti-aging philosophies with the release of this international bestselling book, *The Hot and Sexy Hormone Solution* – for smart and savvy women over 40 aging before their years, a game changing concept for taking "years off" people's age.

With his proprietary Youthful Blueprint System™, Dr. Moricz continues to provide these life changing therapies that have delivered small miracles to his clients, even when nothing else has worked.

Having practiced internationally, Dr. Moricz draws VIP clients from all over the U.S. and even overseas for his therapies. A few things that you may not know about Dr. Moricz is that his VIP clients have fondly named him their "youthful sexuality doctor" and are no longer surprised that he doesn't sugar coat the truth.

Dedicated to Your Body Hormone Transformation,

George Moricz, M.D.

Your Youthful Sexuality Doctor

Concierge Doctor

www.doctormoricz.com

LIVES. CHANGED.

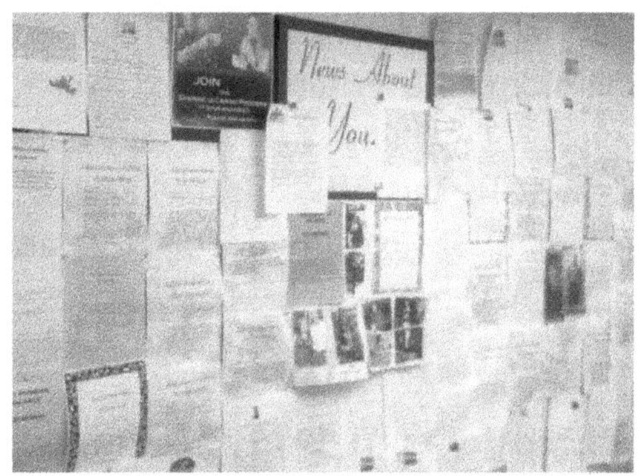

George F. Moricz, MD

Founder of Your Youthful Blueprint